THE COVID-19 PANDEMIC

A Global Crisis Unveiled

BY

DR. MARY I. VERA

DISCLAIMER

TABLE OF CONTENTS

Disclaimer
Introduction
Chapter 1: The Origins and Spread of COVID-19
Chapter 2: Understanding COVID-19
Chapter 3: Prevention and Control Measures
Chapter 4: Health Impacts
Chapter 5: Global Response and Affected Countries
Chapter 6: Lives Lost and Societal Impact
Chapter 7: Economic Consequence
Chapter8: Global Collaboration and Research Efforts
Chapter 9: Mental Health and Social Implications
Chapter 10: Education and Digital Divide
Chapter 11: Lessons Learned and Future Preparedness
Chapter 12: Moving Forward and Building Resilience
Conclusion

INTRODUCTION

The COVID-19 pandemic, caused by the novel coronavirus SARS-CoV-2, has emerged as one of the most significant global health crises in recent history. First identified in December 2019 in Wuhan, China, this infectious disease has rapidly spread across continents, affecting millions of people and leading to profound social, economic, and health consequences. This article delves into the causes, prevention measures, impact on affected countries, lives lost, and the subsequent economic breakdown caused by the COVID-19 pandemic.

CHAPTER 1

The Origins and Spread of COVID-19

The emergence of COVID-19 as a global pandemic can be traced back to its origins in a seafood market in Wuhan, China, in December 2019. The virus, known as SARS-CoV-2, belongs to the family of coronaviruses, which also includes SARS-CoV and MERS-CoV. It is believed to have originated from bats and possibly transmitted to humans through an intermediate animal host.

The initial outbreak in Wuhan quickly escalated into a widespread transmission within the city and soon spread beyond its borders. The high population density, international travel, and globalization played significant roles in the rapid global dissemination of the virus. Infected individuals who traveled internationally unwittingly carried the virus to other countries, sparking outbreaks in various regions.

CHAPTER 2
Understanding COVID-19

COVID-19 primarily spreads through respiratory droplets when an infected person coughs, sneezes, talks, or breathes heavily. The virus can also be transmitted by touching contaminated surfaces and then touching the face, although this is considered a less common route. The incubation period of the virus ranges from 2 to 14 days, during which an infected person may be asymptomatic but still contagious.

Common symptoms of COVID-19 include fever, cough, fatigue, loss of taste or smell, and difficulty breathing. Severe cases can lead to pneumonia and acute respiratory distress syndrome (ARDS). Certain individuals, such as the elderly and those with underlying health conditions like diabetes, hypertension, or compromised immune systems, are more susceptible to severe illness and complications.

Diagnostic methods for COVID-19 include polymerase chain reaction (PCR) tests, which detect the genetic material of the virus, and antigen tests, which identify specific viral proteins. Rapid testing has been crucial in identifying and isolating infected individuals promptly, thus limiting the spread of the virus.

CHAPTER 3

Prevention and Control Measures

Prevention and control measures have been crucial in slowing the transmission of COVID-19. Personal hygiene practices, such as frequent handwashing with soap and water for at least 20 seconds, have been emphasized as a key preventive measure. Wearing masks, particularly in crowded indoor spaces or when social distancing is challenging, has also proven effective in reducing transmission rates.

Social distancing measures, including the closure of schools, businesses, and public gatherings, have been implemented to minimize close contact and mitigate the spread of the virus. Lockdowns and stay-at-home orders have been enforced in many countries to suppress the transmission and relieve pressure on healthcare systems.

Vaccination campaigns have played a vital role in curbing the pandemic. The development and distribution of multiple COVID-19 vaccines, with varying efficacy rates, have been instrumental in reducing the severity of illness, hospitalizations, and deaths. Vaccination efforts have focused on prioritizing high-risk individuals, healthcare workers, and vulnerable populations.

CHAPTER 4

Health Impact

COVID-19 primarily affects the respiratory system, causing a range of respiratory symptoms, including cough, shortness of breath, and pneumonia. However, it has become evident that the impacts of the virus extend beyond the respiratory system. Studies have indicated potential long-term consequences, such as cardiovascular complications, neurological effects, and persistent fatigue, collectively known as "long COVID."

The pandemic has placed immense strain on healthcare systems worldwide. Insufficient hospital beds, medical equipment, and healthcare professionals have challenged the capacity to provide adequate care to all patients. Medical professionals have worked tirelessly, facing high risks of infection and mental health strain due to the demanding circumstances.

The mental health implications of the pandemic have been significant. Isolation, fear, and uncertainty have contributed to increased rates of anxiety, depression, and stress. Access to mental health services has become crucial to support individuals affected by the psychological toll of

CHAPTER 5

Global Response and Affected Countries

The response to the COVID-19 pandemic has varied across countries and regions, reflecting the diversity of healthcare systems, government policies, and societal factors. Some countries implemented strict containment measures early on, including widespread testing, contact tracing, and quarantines. Others faced challenges in effectively implementing and enforcing preventive measures due to logistical constraints or public resistance.

Different countries adopted varying approaches, such as lockdowns, travel restrictions, and border closures, to control the spread of the virus. The success of these measures depended on factors like the timing of implementation, public compliance, and the capacity of healthcare systems to handle the surge in cases.

Disparities in healthcare systems and resources have been evident during the pandemic. Countries with robust healthcare infrastructure and universal access to healthcare fared better in managing the crisis. However, low- and middle-income countries faced significant challenges due to limited resources, inadequate testing capacities, and healthcare infrastructure strains.

The pandemic's impact on affected countries has been profound. It has disrupted economies, strained public health systems, and challenged social cohesion. Some countries experienced higher mortality rates and overwhelmed healthcare systems, leading to difficult decisions about resource allocation and triage. The availability of vaccines and access to healthcare resources have also been unevenly distributed, exacerbating global health inequalities.

Additionally, the pandemic has exposed vulnerabilities in sectors like education, transportation, tourism, and retail. Schools and universities faced closures, leading to disruptions in learning and impacting students' academic progress. The tourism industry, which heavily relies on international travel, experienced a sharp decline, resulting in job losses and economic downturns in many countries.

The economic consequences of the pandemic have been severe. Businesses, especially small and medium enterprises, struggled to survive amid lockdowns and reduced consumer spending. Unemployment rates soared as companies downsized or shut down operations. Governments implemented various fiscal and monetary policies to mitigate the economic impact, including stimulus packages, loans, and financial assistance programs.

In conclusion, the COVID-19 pandemic has revealed the interconnectedness of our global society and the importance of a coordinated, science-driven response to public health emergencies. The understanding of COVID-19, along with preventive measures like personal hygiene, social distancing, and vaccination, has been crucial in controlling the spread of the virus. However, the pandemic has also exposed weaknesses in healthcare systems, highlighted social and economic disparities, and emphasized the need for international collaboration to address future pandemics effectively. Moving forward, it is essential to learn from this experience, strengthen healthcare infrastructure, and prioritize equitable access to healthcare and resources for all

CHAPTER 6

Lives Lost and Societal Impact

The COVID-19 pandemic has exacted a devastating toll on human lives. Millions of individuals have lost their lives to the virus, leaving families and communities grieving. The elderly and those with underlying health conditions have been particularly vulnerable, with higher mortality rates observed among these populations. The loss of lives has not only brought immense sorrow but also significant social and emotional consequences for affected families and communities.

The impact of the pandemic extends beyond the loss of lives. It has disrupted daily life routines and social interactions on a global scale. Lockdowns and stay-at-home orders have resulted in isolation, loneliness, and mental health challenges for many individuals. The closure of schools and educational institutions has disrupted learning, affecting the academic progress and social development of students.

Furthermore, the pandemic has highlighted and exacerbated existing social and economic inequalities. Marginalized communities, including racial and ethnic minorities, low-income individuals, and migrants, have faced disproportionate impacts. Limited access to healthcare, higher rates of comorbidities, and economic vulnerabilities have contributed to higher infection rates and poorer health outcomes among these populations.

CHAPTER 7

Economic Consequences

The COVID-19 pandemic has triggered a severe global economic crisis. Lockdowns, travel restrictions, and the closure of businesses have led to an unprecedented downturn in various sectors. Industries such as tourism, hospitality, retail, and entertainment have been particularly hard-hit, experiencing substantial revenue losses and widespread layoffs.

The pandemic-induced economic crisis has resulted in increased unemployment rates worldwide. Many businesses, especially small and medium enterprises, have struggled to survive, leading to job losses and financial instability for millions of workers. Governments have implemented fiscal stimulus packages and financial assistance programs to support businesses and individuals, but the road to recovery remains challenging.

Global supply chains have also been disrupted due to restrictions on trade and transportation. This has affected industries reliant on imports and exports, leading to shortages of essential goods and raw materials. The economic interdependencies among nations have exposed vulnerabilities, highlighting the need for resilient and diversified supply chains.

Government responses to the economic crisis have varied, with interventions ranging from direct cash transfers, loan programs, and wage subsidies to prevent widespread bankruptcies and alleviate financial distress. Central banks have implemented monetary policies such as interest rate cuts and quantitative easing to stimulate economic activity and maintain financial stability.

The long-term economic impact of the pandemic remains uncertain. The recovery process is expected to be gradual, with some sectors rebounding faster than others. The distribution of vaccines and the ability to achieve widespread vaccination coverage will play a crucial role in restoring consumer confidence, reopening economies, and reigniting growth.

CHAPTER 8

Global Collaboration and Research Efforts

The global nature of the COVID-19 pandemic has necessitated unprecedented levels of collaboration among scientists, researchers, and healthcare professionals worldwide. International organizations, such as the World Health Organization (WHO), have played a central role in coordinating efforts, providing guidance, and sharing information.

Research efforts have been accelerated to better understand the virus, its variants, and the development of effective treatments and vaccines. Scientists have collaborated to sequence the viral genome, study its transmission dynamics, and investigate potential therapeutics. International clinical trials have been conducted to evaluate the safety and efficacy of various treatment options, contributing to the evolving understanding of COVID-19 management.

Additionally, the development of vaccines has been a remarkable achievement in a short period. Global cooperation has been essential in the rapid development, testing, and distribution of multiple vaccines. Collaborative initiatives, such as COVAX, have aimed to ensure equitable access to vaccines for all countries, particularly low- and middle-income nations.

CHAPTER 9
Mental Health and Social Implications

The COVID-19 pandemic has had profound effects on mental health and social well-being. The prolonged period of uncertainty, fear, and social isolation has resulted in increased levels of anxiety, depression, and stress. The mental health impacts have been felt across all age groups, with particular vulnerabilities among frontline healthcare workers, children, and individuals with pre-existing mental health conditions.

Access to mental health services and support has become crucial during these challenging times. Teletherapy, online counseling, and helplines have been utilized to provide remote mental health support. Governments and organizations have implemented awareness campaigns and initiatives to reduce stigma, promote self-care, and facilitate access to mental health resources.

The pandemic has also exposed social inequalities and highlighted the importance of social cohesion. Vulnerable populations, including the homeless, refugees, and marginalized communities, have faced increased hardships, limited access to healthcare, and economic disparities. Community support networks and initiatives have been vital in addressing these inequalities and providing assistance to those most in need.

CHAPTER 10
Education and Digital Divide

The closure of schools and educational institutions during the pandemic has significantly disrupted learning and highlighted existing disparities in access to education. The shift to remote learning has posed challenges for students, teachers, and parents, particularly in regions with limited internet connectivity and technology resources.

The digital divide has become more evident, with disadvantaged students facing difficulties in accessing online classes and resources. Efforts have been made to bridge this gap through initiatives such as providing devices and internet access to students in need. However, the digital divide remains a significant hurdle in ensuring equitable education during the pandemic.

Educational systems have had to adapt to the new normal, implementing hybrid learning models, virtual classrooms, and innovative teaching methods. Teachers have faced the challenge of engaging students remotely, while students have grappled with adjusting to virtual learning environments and maintaining motivation.

CHAPTER 11

Lessons Learned and Future Preparedness

The COVID-19 pandemic has provided valuable lessons for governments, healthcare systems, and societies worldwide. It has exposed vulnerabilities in global preparedness for pandemics and highlighted the importance of proactive measures, early detection, and rapid response.

Investments in public health infrastructure, including surveillance systems, testing capabilities, and healthcare workforce training, are crucial for early detection and containment of future outbreaks. International collaboration and information sharing should be further strengthened to facilitate a coordinated response and prevent the spread of infectious diseases across borders.

Pandemic preparedness plans should prioritize the equitable distribution of essential resources, including vaccines, medical supplies, and personal protective equipment. Investments in research and development, particularly in antiviral treatments and vaccine production technologies, are necessary to enhance global readiness for future health emergencies.

CHAPTER 12
Moving Forward and Building Resilience

As the world continues to navigate the challenges of the COVID-19 pandemic, it is crucial to focus on building resilience and preparing for future health crises. This involves implementing strategies that encompass various aspects of society, including healthcare, economy, education, and social well-being.

In the healthcare sector, investments should be made to strengthen healthcare systems, improve diagnostic capabilities, and expand vaccine manufacturing capacities. Building robust public health infrastructure and surveillance systems can enhance early detection and response to potential outbreaks. Research and development in virology, immunology, and epidemiology should be prioritized to better understand emerging infectious diseases and develop effective preventive and therapeutic interventions.

Economically, countries need to diversify their industries and supply chains to reduce dependence on a single sector or region. Promoting innovation, entrepreneurship, and small business support can enhance economic resilience. Governments should also focus on social safety nets, job retraining programs, and economic recovery measures to mitigate the impact of future crises on vulnerable populations.

Education systems must adapt to be more resilient in the face of disruptions. This includes incorporating digital learning tools and infrastructure, ensuring access to quality education for all students, and enhancing teacher training for remote and hybrid teaching methods. Close collaboration between governments, educators, and technology providers is essential to bridge the digital divide and ensure equitable access to education.

Addressing mental health and social well-being should also be a priority. Governments and communities must continue to promote mental health awareness and provide accessible mental health services. Social support networks and community engagement programs should be strengthened to foster resilience and social cohesion in times of crisis.

International collaboration and cooperation remain vital in managing global health emergencies. Governments, organizations, and researchers must continue to share knowledge, data, and resources to respond effectively to future outbreaks. Strengthening partnerships between countries and investing in global health governance can improve preparedness and facilitate a coordinated response in times of crisis.

In conclusion, the COVID-19 pandemic has been a wake-up call, emphasizing the need for preparedness, resilience, and global collaboration in the face of health crises. By applying the lessons learned from this pandemic, societies can build stronger healthcare systems, more robust economies, inclusive education systems, and enhanced mental health support networks. It is through these collective efforts that we can better navigate future challenges and protect the well-being of individuals and communities worldwide.

CONCLUSION

The COVID-19 pandemic has underscored the importance of global collaboration, effective healthcare systems, and robust preventive measures. It has exposed vulnerabilities in public health infrastructure worldwide and prompted the scientific community to accelerate research and development efforts. As countries continue to battle the virus, the lessons learned from this crisis should serve as a reminder of the need for preparedness, resilience, and international cooperation to mitigate the impact of future pandemics.